PLANT BASED DIET COOKBOOK FOR BEGINNERS 2024

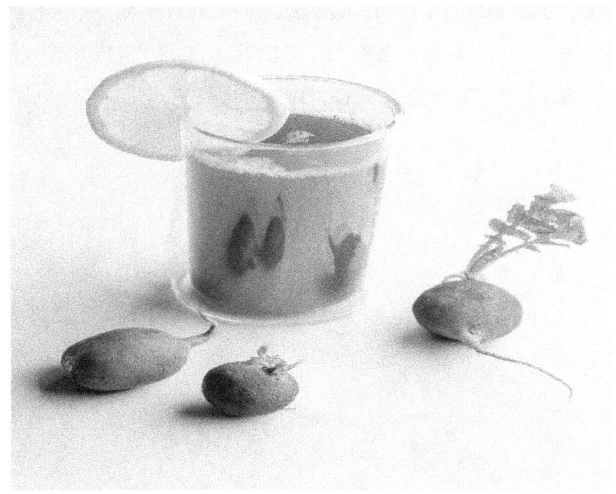

Quick, Easy and Tasty Recipes to Create a Balanced Lifestyle within 30 Days

Nora Bolton

Table Of Content

CHAPTER ONE

1 INTRODUCTION

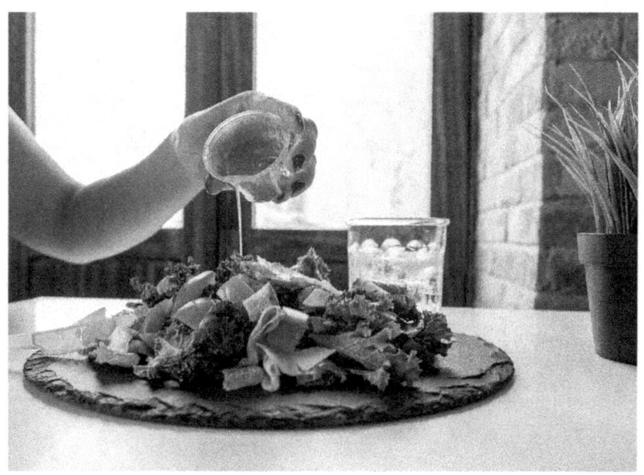

In the vibrant heart of Green Valley, where lush fields and towering forests met, a quiet revolution was taking root. The residents of this idyllic community had embraced a transformative way of life — the Plant-Based Diet. The story unfolded with a farmer named Nora, who, with soil-stained hands and a heart full of purpose, had pioneered this movement.

Nora's journey began when she discovered the profound impact of plant-based living on personal health and the environment. With unwavering determination, she cultivated a diverse array of fruits, vegetables, and legumes on her farm, educating her neighbors about the boundless benefits of embracing nature's bounty.

The aroma of roasted vegetables and the sizzle of plant-based burgers filled the air as Green Valley's inhabitants gathered for communal meals, celebrating the flavors that sprang forth from the earth. A sense of vitality and unity permeated the town, and as the once skeptical inhabitants tasted the richness of this lifestyle, they became fervent advocates.

In the heart of Green Valley, a once-neglected community garden bloomed into a thriving hub of sustainable living. Farmers' markets bustled with vibrant colors and lively chatter, showcasing the variety of produce that now flourished in abundance. The rhythm of life in Green Valley had harmonized with the rhythm of the natural world.

As news of Green Valley's plant-based revolution spread, neighboring communities took notice. The movement sparked conversations about mindful consumption, ecological responsibility, and a reconnection with the land. People from distant places visited, eager to learn the secrets of Green Valley's vitality.

Nora's farm became a symbol of hope, a testament to the transformative power of a plant-based lifestyle. The once-skeptical townsfolk found themselves healthier, more energetic, and deeply connected to the environment. In the quiet fields of Green Valley, a verdant legacy grew, weaving together the stories of individuals, a community, and a planet on the path to renewal.

1.1 Understanding the plant based diet

A plant-based diet revolves around consuming foods derived primarily from plants, such as fruits, vegetables, grains, nuts, and seeds, while minimizing or eliminating animal products. This dietary choice has gained significant attention for its potential health benefits and its positive impact on the environment.

From a nutritional perspective, a well-balanced plant-based diet can provide essential vitamins, minerals, fiber, and antioxidants. Fruits and vegetables are rich in micronutrients that contribute to overall well-being and may reduce the risk of chronic diseases. Additionally, plant-based diets often have lower levels of saturated fat and cholesterol, potentially promoting heart health.

Environmental sustainability is a driving force behind the adoption of plant-based diets. Animal agriculture is resource-intensive, requiring vast amounts of land, water, and energy. Choosing plant-based options can reduce the ecological footprint associated with food production, helping to mitigate climate change and preserve biodiversity.

Moreover, ethical considerations play a role in the decision to adopt a plant-based lifestyle. Some individuals choose this diet to align with their values related to animal welfare, as plant-based diets typically involve less harm to animals compared to conventional omnivorous diets.

However, it's crucial to approach a plant-based diet mindfully to ensure adequate nutrient intake. Certain nutrients like vitamin B12, iron, and omega-3 fatty acids may require special attention and supplementation.

In conclusion, understanding the plant-based diet involves recognizing its diverse benefits, from potential health advantages to environmental sustainability and ethical considerations. While adopting such a diet can be a positive choice, it's important to plan meals carefully to meet nutritional needs effectively.

1.2 **Benefits of adopting a plant based diet**

Adopting a plant-based diet offers a myriad of benefits for both individuals and the environment. Firstly, it promotes overall health by reducing the risk of chronic diseases such as heart disease, diabetes, and certain types of cancer. Plant-based diets are rich in fiber, vitamins, and antioxidants while being lower in saturated fats and cholesterol, contributing to better weight management and improved blood sugar levels.

Moreover, a plant-based diet supports environmental sustainability. Livestock farming is a major contributor to deforestation, greenhouse gas emissions, and water pollution. By choosing plant-based options, individuals contribute to reducing their carbon footprint, preserving biodiversity, and conserving water resources. The production of plant-based foods generally requires less land and water compared to raising livestock, making it a more eco-friendly choice.

Embracing a plant-based lifestyle can also enhance ethical considerations. Many people adopt this diet due to concerns about animal welfare, as the industrial farming practices associated with meat production often involve inhumane conditions for animals. Choosing plant-based alternatives aligns with a compassionate approach towards animals, fostering a more ethical and humane food system.

In conclusion, a plant-based diet is a holistic choice that not only promotes personal well-being but also addresses environmental and ethical considerations. Making conscious food choices towards plant-based options can contribute to a healthier, more sustainable, and compassionate world.

1.3 Getting Started

Embarking on a plant-based diet requires several key steps to ensure a smooth transition into this nutrient-rich lifestyle focused on plant-derived foods.

Educate Yourself: Begin by understanding the principles of a plant-based diet. Learn about the benefits, nutritional requirements, and potential challenges. Resources like documentaries, books, and reputable websites can provide valuable information.

Gradual Transition: Instead of making abrupt changes, consider a gradual transition. Start by incorporating more fruits, vegetables, whole grains, and legumes into your meals. Replace meat with plant-based protein sources like tofu, beans, and lentils.

Explore New Recipes: Experiment with plant-based recipes to discover delicious and satisfying meals. There are countless online resources, cookbooks, and apps dedicated to plant-based cooking. Get creative in the kitchen to make the transition enjoyable.

Balanced Nutrition: Ensure a well-rounded diet by including a variety of foods. Pay attention to getting an adequate amount of protein, vitamins, and minerals. Consider consulting a nutritionist or using apps to track your nutrient intake initially.

Read Labels: Be mindful of food labels to identify hidden animal products. Some processed foods may contain ingredients like dairy or gelatin. Familiarize yourself with plant-based alternatives for common ingredients.

Stay Hydrated: Water is crucial for overall health. Drink an ample amount of water daily to stay hydrated. Herbal teas and plant-based milk alternatives can also be good options.

Plan Meals: Plan your meals and snacks in advance to ensure you have a variety of plant-based options readily available. This can help prevent resorting to less healthy choices when hungry.

Supplements: Consider consulting a healthcare professional to determine if you need any supplements, such as vitamin B12 or omega-3 fatty acids, which can be less abundant in a plant-based diet.

Community Support: Connect with others who follow a plant-based lifestyle. Online forums, social media groups, or local meetups can provide valuable support, tips, and motivation.

Listen to Your Body: Pay attention to how your body responds to the changes. If needed, make adjustments to your diet to meet your individual nutritional requirements.

Remember, adopting a plant-based diet is a personal journey, and finding what works best for you is key.

CHAPTER TWO

2 30 Day Meal Plan

A 30-day meal plan is a structured guide outlining daily meals for a month. It typically includes breakfast, lunch, dinner, and snacks, aiming to provide a balanced and nutritious diet. These plans can be tailored for various goals, such as weight loss, muscle gain, or overall health improvement. They often include portion control, diverse food choices, and specific recipes to help individuals achieve their dietary objectives over the designated time frame.

2.1 Week 1: meal plan for day 1-7 recipes

Day 1:

- Breakfast: spinach-filled scrambled eggs and wholegrain bread

- Lunch: mixed veggie and vinaigrette dressing grilled chicken salad

- Dinner: Baked salmon with quinoa and roasted asparagus

Day 2:

- Breakfast: Berries with Greek yogurt with a honey drizzle

- Lunch: Quinoa and black bean bowl with salsa and avocado

- Dinner: Stir-fried tofu with broccoli and brown rice

Day 3:

- Breakfast: Oatmeal with sliced banana and almond butter

- Lunch: Whole wheat tortilla wrap with turkey and vegetables

- Dinner: Lemon herb grilled shrimp with sweet potato wedges and green beans

Day 4:

- Breakfast: Whole grain waffles with fresh strawberries and yogurt

- Lunch: Brown rice and vegetable and chickpea curry

- Dinner: Beef stir-fry with bell peppers and snap peas over noodles

Day 5:

- Breakfast: spinach, banana, almond milk, and protein powder blended into a smoothie

- Lunch: Caprese salad with whole grain crackers

- Dinner: Grilled swordfish with quinoa and steamed broccoli

Day 6:

- Breakfast: Avocado toast with cherry tomatoes and a sprinkle of feta cheese

- Lunch: Served with a serving of mixed greens, lentil soup

- Dinner: Roasted chicken breast with sweet potato mash and green beans

Day 7:

- Breakfast: Cottage cheese with pineapple chunks and a handful of nuts

- Lunch: Whole grain pasta with marinara sauce, grilled vegetables, and Parmesan cheese

- Dinner: Vegetarian chili with cornbread on the side

Explanation:

These meal ideas provide a balance of protein, carbohydrates, and healthy fats.
Lean protein options include fish, poultry, tofu, and lentils.
Include a variety of colorful vegetables to ensure a good mix of vitamins and minerals.
Whole grains like quinoa, brown rice, and whole wheat contribute complex carbohydrates.
Healthy fats can come from sources like avocados, nuts, and olive oil.
Don't forget to stay hydrated throughout the day with water or herbal teas.
Feel free to adjust portion sizes based on individual needs and dietary preferences.

2.2 **Week 2: meal plan for day 8-14 Recipes**

Day 8:

- Breakfast: Avocado Toast

Ingredients:
Whole grain bread
Avocado
Cherry tomatoes
Olive oil
Salt and pepper
Instructions: Toast the bread, mash the avocado, spread it on the toast, and top with sliced cherry tomatoes.Add a drizzle of olive oil and season with pepper and salt.

- Lunch: Quinoa Salad

Ingredients:
Quinoa
Mixed vegetables (bell peppers, cucumber, red onion)
Feta cheese
Lemon vinaigrette dressing
Instructions: Cook quinoa, mix with chopped vegetables and feta cheese. Toss with lemon vinaigrette dressing.

- Dinner: Grilled Chicken with Sweet Potato

Ingredients:
Chicken breast
Sweet potatoes
Olive oil
Garlic powder, paprika, salt, and pepper
Instructions: Season chicken with spices, grill until cooked. Roast sweet potato wedges with olive oil, salt, and pepper.

Day 9-14:

Repeat a similar pattern with variations. For example:

Day 9:

- Breakfast: Greek Yogurt Parfait

- Lunch: Lentil Soup with Whole Grain Roll

- Dinner: Baked Salmon with Asparagus

Day 10:

- Breakfast: Oatmeal with Berries and Almonds

- Lunch: Chickpea Salad Wrap

- Dinner: Vegetable Stir-Fry with Brown Rice

Continue with a diverse mix of proteins, whole grains, and colorful vegetables throughout the week, ensuring a balance of nutrients. Adjust portion sizes based on personal dietary needs and goals.

Explanation:

Variety: This plan includes a variety of nutrient-dense foods to ensure you get a wide range of essential nutrients.
Balance: Each meal combines protein, healthy fats, and carbohydrates for balanced nutrition.
Customization: Feel free to adjust quantities and ingredients based on your preferences and dietary requirements.
Remember to stay hydrated, listen to your body's hunger and fullness cues, and adapt the plan to suit your individual needs and preferences

2.3 Week 3: meal plan for day 15-21 Recipes

Day 15:

- Breakfast: Scrambled Eggs with Spinach and Feta

Ingredients: Eggs, fresh spinach, feta cheese
Instructions: Scramble eggs, sauté spinach, mix with eggs, add crumbled feta.

- Lunch: Quinoa Salad with Roasted Vegetables

Ingredients: Quinoa, mixed vegetables (bell peppers, zucchini, cherry tomatoes), olive oil
Instructions: Cook quinoa, roast vegetables, toss together with olive oil.

- Dinner: Baked Lemon Herb Chicken

Ingredients: Chicken breasts, lemon, herbs (rosemary, thyme), olive oil
Instructions: Marinate chicken in lemon and herbs, bake until cooked through.

Day 16:

- Breakfast: Greek Yogurt Parfait

Ingredients: Greek yogurt, granola, mixed berries
Instructions: Layer Greek yogurt, granola, and berries in a glass.

- Lunch: Chickpea and Vegetable Stir-Fry

Ingredients: Chickpeas, broccoli, carrots, soy sauce
Instructions: Stir-fry chickpeas and veggies with soy sauce.

- Dinner: Salmon with Garlic Butter and
  Asparagus

Ingredients: Salmon filets, garlic, butter, asparagus
Instructions: Sear salmon, cook asparagus, make
garlic butter, drizzle over salmon.

Day 17:

- Breakfast: Oatmeal with Banana and
  Almonds

Ingredients: Oats, banana slices, almonds
Instructions: Cook oats, top with banana slices and
almonds.

- Lunch: Lentil Soup

Ingredients: Lentils, carrots, celery, vegetable broth
Instructions: Cook lentils and veggies in vegetable
broth.

- Dinner: Turkey and Vegetable Skewers

Ingredients: Turkey chunks, bell peppers, red onion,
olive oil
Instructions: Skewer turkey and veggies, grill or
bake until cooked.

Day 18:

- Breakfast: Whole Wheat Toast with Avocado

Ingredients: Whole wheat bread, avocado, salt,
pepper
Instructions: Toast bread, spread avocado, sprinkle
with salt and pepper.

- Lunch: Spinach and Mushroom Quesadillas
Ingredients: Flour tortillas, spinach, mushrooms,
cheese
Instructions: Fill tortillas with sautéed spinach,
mushrooms, and cheese, cook until cheese melts.

- Dinner: Beef and Broccoli Stir-Fry
Ingredients: Beef strips, broccoli, soy sauce, ginger
Instructions: Stir-fry beef and broccoli with soy
sauce and ginger.

Day 19-21:

Feel free to mix and match from the previous days
or repeat any favorites. This provides variety while
maintaining a balanced meal plan.
Explanation:
Each meal includes a good balance of protein,
carbohydrates, and healthy fats.
Incorporating a variety of vegetables ensures a
range of nutrients.
Portion sizes should be adjusted based on individual
dietary needs and goals.

Hydration with water and herbal teas is important throughout the day.

Remember, this is a general guideline, and you can customize it based on personal preferences and dietary restrictions.

2.4 **Week 4: meal plan for day 22-30 Recipes**

Day 22:

- Breakfast: Avocado Toast with Poached Eggs
    - Whole-grain toast topped with mashed avocado and poached eggs.
- Lunch: Quinoa Salad Bowl
    - Quinoa mixed with colorful vegetables, chickpeas, and a lemon-tahini dressing.
- Dinner: Baked Lemon Herb Chicken
    - Chicken breasts seasoned with herbs and baked with lemon, served with roasted sweet potatoes and steamed broccoli.

Day 23:

- Breakfast: Greek Yogurt Parfait

- Greek yogurt layered with fresh berries, granola, and a drizzle of honey.
- **Lunch: Turkey and Vegetable Wrap**
  - Whole-grain wrap filled with lean turkey, mixed greens, tomatoes, and hummus.
- **Dinner: Vegetarian Stir-Fry**
  - Tofu or tempeh stir-fried with a variety of colorful vegetables in a soy-ginger sauce, served over brown rice.

Day 24:

- **Breakfast: Spinach and Feta Omelette**
  - Omelet with sautéed spinach and feta cheese.
- **Lunch: Chickpea Salad**
  - Chickpeas mixed with cucumber, cherry tomatoes, feta, and a balsamic vinaigrette.
- **Dinner: Grilled Salmon with Quinoa**
  - Grilled salmon filets served with lemon-dill quinoa and steamed asparagus.

Continue this pattern for the remaining days, incorporating a mix of lean proteins, whole grains, and plenty of vegetables for balanced nutrition. Adjust portion sizes based on individual dietary needs and preferences.

Remember to stay hydrated throughout the day and consider incorporating healthy snacks like fruits, nuts, or yogurt between meals for sustained energy.

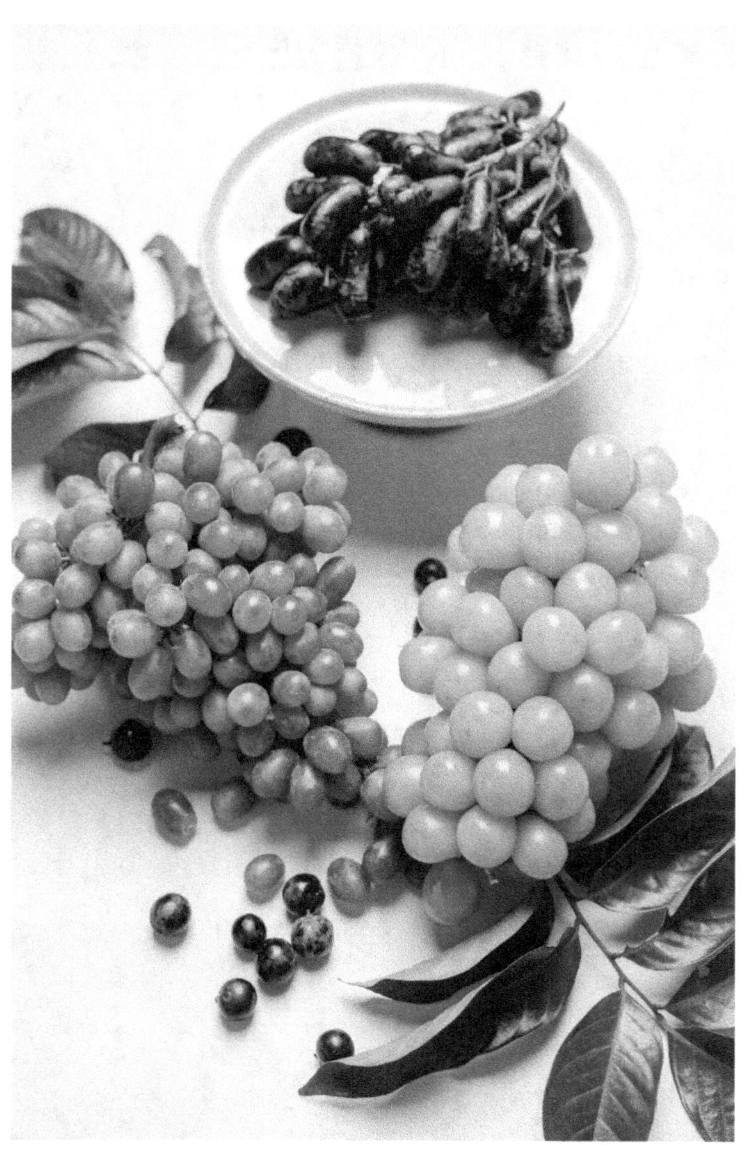

CHAPTER THREE

3 Quick and Easy Recipes

Quick and easy recipes in a plant-based diet refer to meal preparations that are not only simple and efficient but also align with the principles of plant-based eating. These recipes typically focus on using whole, plant-based ingredients to create flavorful and nutritious dishes without extensive cooking time or complicated techniques. Now, let's explore some examples of quick and easy plant-based recipes.

3.1 Smoothies and breakfast

Smoothie Recipe: Berry Blast

Ingredients:

1 cup mixed berries (strawberries, blueberries, raspberries)
1 banana
1/2 cup Greek yogurt
1/2 cup almond milk
1 tablespoon honey
Ice cubes (optional)
Instructions:

Blend all ingredients until smooth.
Add ice cubes if desired for a colder texture.
Pour into a glass and enjoy your berry blast
smoothie!
Breakfast Recipe: Avocado Toast

Ingredients:

1 slice whole-grain bread
1 ripe avocado
Salt and pepper to taste
Optional toppings: cherry tomatoes, red pepper
flakes, poached egg
Instructions:

Toast the whole-grain bread slice.
Spread the mashed, ripe avocado on top of the
toast.
Add a dash of pepper and salt.
Add your favorite toppings, such as cherry tomatoes
or a poached egg.
Enjoy a quick and nutritious avocado toast for
breakfast!

3.2 Sweets

No-Bake Chocolate Peanut Butter Bars:

Ingredients:

1 cup creamy peanut butter
1/2 cup unsalted butter, melted
2 cups powdered sugar
2 cups graham cracker crumbs
1 1/2 cups chocolate chips
1 tablespoon vegetable oil

Instructions:

In a bowl, mix peanut butter, melted butter,
powdered sugar, and graham cracker crumbs until
well combined.
Press the mixture evenly into a lined square baking
pan.
In a microwave-safe bowl, melt chocolate chips with
vegetable oil in 30-second intervals, stirring until
smooth.
Pour the melted chocolate over the peanut butter
layer and spread it evenly.
Chill for a minimum of two hours or until solidified,
cut into squares and enjoy your no-bake chocolate
peanut butter bars!

Garlic Parmesan Roasted Broccoli:
Toss broccoli florets with olive oil, minced garlic, and grated Parmesan.
Bake until crispy.

Caprese Skewers:
Put fresh mozzarella, cherry tomatoes, and basil leaves on skewers.
Drizzle with balsamic glaze.

Avocado Toast with a Twist:
Spread mashed avocado on whole-grain toast.
Top with cherry tomatoes, feta cheese, and a sprinkle of chili flakes.

Sweet Potato Fries:
Cut sweet potatoes into fries, coat with olive oil and season with paprika and salt.
Bake until golden and crispy.

Hummus and Veggie Platter:
Arrange cucumber slices, carrot sticks, and cherry tomatoes on a platter.
Serve with your favorite hummus.

Guacamole with Pita Chips:

Mash avocados, mix with diced tomatoes, onions,
lime juice, and salt.
Accompany with warm pita chips.

Greek Yogurt Dip:
Mix Greek yogurt with minced garlic, dill, and lemon
juice.
Perfect for dipping veggies or whole-grain crackers.

Crispy Kale Chips:
Toss kale leaves with olive oil, salt, and pepper.
Bake until crispy for a healthy snack.

Stuffed Mushrooms:
Fill mushroom caps with a mixture of cream cheese,
garlic, and herbs.
Bake until the mushrooms are tender.

Fruit Salad with Mint:
Combine fresh fruit chunks and toss with chopped
mint.
Drizzle with honey for a refreshing side or snack.

3.4 Main courses

One-Pan Chicken and Vegetables:
Toss chicken breasts, potatoes, and your favorite
veggies with olive oil and seasonings.
Bake for 25 to 30 minutes at 400°F (200°C).

Pasta Aglio e Olio:
Cook spaghetti, sauté minced garlic in olive oil, add
red pepper flakes.
Toss cooked pasta in the garlic oil, add parsley, and
a squeeze of lemon.

Sheet Pan Fajitas:
Mix sliced bell peppers, onions, and chicken strips
with fajita seasoning.
Roast on a sheet pan at 425°F (220°C) for 20-25
minutes.

Quick Stir-Fry:
Stir-fry your choice of protein (chicken, beef, tofu)
with colorful veggies.
Add soy sauce, ginger, and garlic for flavor.

Caprese Chicken:
Top chicken breasts with tomato slices, mozzarella,
and basil.
Bake until chicken is cooked through, then drizzle
with balsamic glaze.

Easy Shrimp Scampi:
Sauté shrimp in butter, garlic, and lemon juice.
Serve with cooked rice or spaghetti.

Homemade Margherita Pizza:

Spread pizza dough with tomato sauce, fresh mozzarella, and basil.
Bake until the cheese is bubbling and the crust is brown.

Teriyaki Salmon:
Marinate salmon filets in teriyaki sauce.
Grill or bake until salmon is flaky.

Spinach and Feta Stuffed Chicken Breast:
Butterfly chicken breasts, stuff with spinach and feta, then bake.

Vegetarian Quesadillas:
Layer black beans, cheese, and veggies between tortillas.
Cook on a skillet until the cheese is melted.
Enjoy these quick and delicious main course recipes!

3.5 Handhelds and Hearty Bowls

Handheld: Turkey Avocado Wrap
Ingredients: Whole wheat tortilla, sliced turkey, avocado, lettuce, tomato, and mayo.

Instructions: Lay out the tortilla, layer turkey slices, add sliced avocado, lettuce, tomato, and a drizzle of mayo. Enjoy it after rolling it up!

Hearty Bowl: Quinoa Veggie Bowl
Ingredients: Cooked quinoa, roasted vegetables (bell peppers, zucchini, carrots), chickpeas, feta cheese, and a lemon-tahini dressing.
Instructions: Mix quinoa with roasted veggies and chickpeas in a bowl. Top with crumbled feta and drizzle the lemon-tahini dressing.

Handheld: Caprese Sandwich
Ingredients: Baguette slices, fresh mozzarella, tomato slices, fresh basil leaves, balsamic glaze.
Instructions: Layer mozzarella, tomato, and basil on baguette slices. Drizzle with balsamic glaze and sandwich together.

Hearty Bowl: Chicken and Rice Bowl
Ingredients: Cooked brown rice, grilled chicken strips, sautéed spinach, cherry tomatoes, and a garlic-lemon sauce.
Instructions: Combine rice, grilled chicken, sautéed spinach, and halved cherry tomatoes in a bowl. Drizzle with garlic-lemon sauce.

Handheld: Veggie Hummus Wrap

Ingredients: Whole grain wrap, hummus, cucumber, bell peppers, shredded carrots, and spinach.
Instructions: Spread hummus on the wrap, layer cucumber, bell peppers, shredded carrots, and spinach. Roll it up for a flavorful veggie wrap.

Hearty Bowl: Beef and Broccoli Rice Bowl
Ingredients: Stir-fried beef strips, broccoli florets, cooked jasmine rice, soy sauce, and sesame oil.
Instructions: Mix stir-fried beef and broccoli with cooked rice. Drizzle with a mixture of soy sauce and sesame oil.
Enjoy these quick and easy handhelds and hearty bowls!

3.6 Staples, Dressings and Condiments

Staples: One-Pot Chickpea and Vegetable Stew

Ingredients:

1 can chickpeas, drained and rinsed
1 cup diced carrots
1 cup diced potatoes
1 cup chopped tomatoes
1 onion, finely chopped
2 cloves garlic, minced
4 cups vegetable broth

1 teaspoon cumin
1 teaspoon paprika
Salt and pepper to taste
Olive oil
Instructions:

In a pot, sauté onions and garlic in olive oil until
softened.
Add carrots, potatoes, and tomatoes. Cook for 5
minutes.
Pour in chickpeas, vegetable broth, cumin, paprika,
salt, and pepper.
Bring to a boil, then simmer for 20-25 minutes until
vegetables are tender.
Serve hot.

Dressings: Honey Mustard Vinaigrette

Ingredients:

3 tablespoons Dijon mustard
2 tablespoons honey
1/4 cup apple cider vinegar
1/2 cup olive oil
Salt and pepper to taste
Instructions:

In a bowl, whisk together Dijon mustard, honey, and
apple cider vinegar.

Slowly drizzle in olive oil while whisking to emulsify.
Season with salt and pepper to taste.
Store in a jar and shake before use.

Condiments: Easy Homemade Salsa

Ingredients:

4 ripe tomatoes, diced
1/2 red onion, finely chopped
1 jalapeño, seeds removed and minced
1/4 cup fresh cilantro, chopped
2 tablespoons lime juice
Salt to taste
Instructions:

Combine tomatoes, red onion, jalapeño, and cilantro
in a bowl.
Stir thoroughly after adding the lime juice.
Season with salt to taste.
Chill for a minimum of half an hour prior to serving.
These recipes are simple, quick, and versatile for
everyday meals. Enjoy!

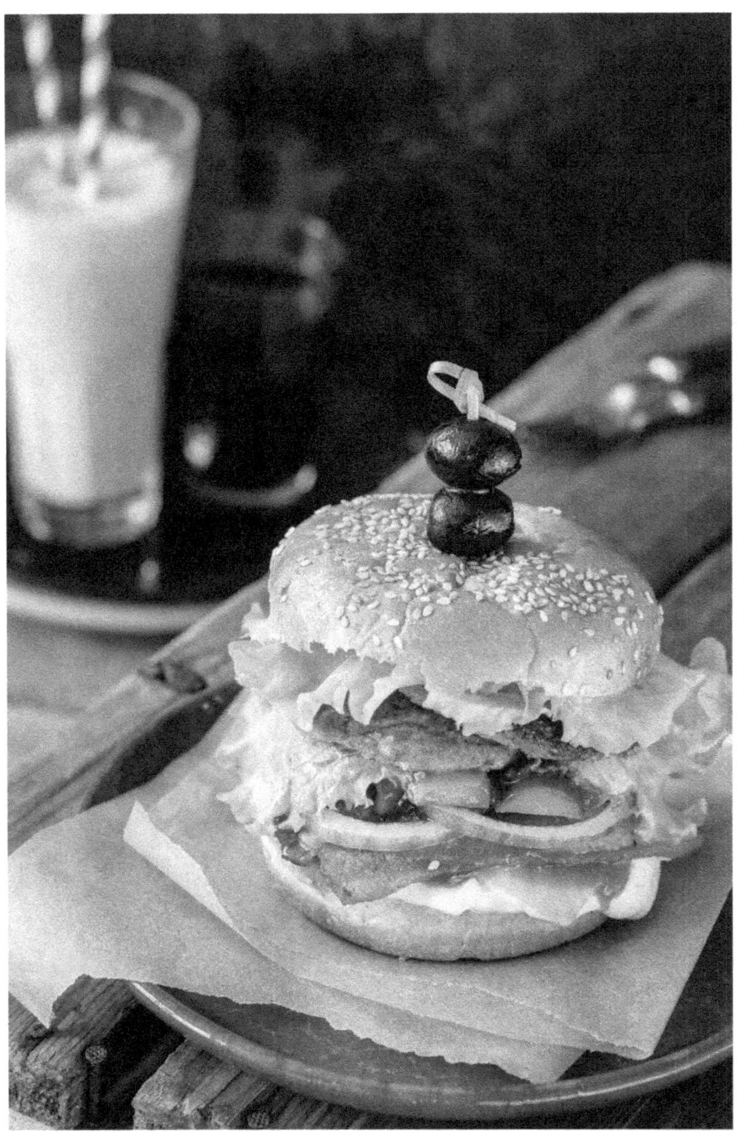

CHAPTER FOUR

4 Tips and Tricks

Tips and tricks in a plant-based diet refer to practical insights and strategies that can help individuals navigate and enhance their experience with plant-based eating. These insights may include ways to optimize nutrition, simplify meal preparation, overcome challenges, and make the transition to a plant-based lifestyle more enjoyable and sustainable. Now, let's explore some useful tips and tricks for a plant-based diet.

4.1 Grocery shopping for a plant based diet

Plan Your Meals: Outline your meals for the week to ensure you have a well-balanced plant-based diet.

Make a Shopping List: Based on your meal plan, create a detailed shopping list to avoid impulse buys.

Explore the Produce Section: Load up on colorful fruits and vegetables for essential vitamins and minerals.

Bulk Up on Legumes: Beans, lentils, and chickpeas are excellent sources of protein and fiber – buy them in bulk to save money.

Whole Grains Are Key: Opt for whole grains like quinoa, brown rice, and oats for a nutrient-rich base.

Nuts and Seeds: Stock up on nuts and seeds for healthy fats and added protein – great for snacking or as toppings.

Plant-Based Protein Alternatives: Explore tofu, tempeh, and plant-based protein sources to diversify your meals.

Check Labels: Be mindful of processed foods; read labels to avoid hidden animal products and excessive additives.

Explore Plant-Based Milk: Try different plant-based milk alternatives like almond, soy, or oat milk.

Frozen Fruits and Vegetables: Convenient and nutritious, these can be used in smoothies, stir-fries, or as sides.

Herbs and Spices: Enhance flavors without relying on animal products – experiment with various herbs and spices.

Meal Prep Essentials: Invest in reusable containers for batch cooking and storing prepared meals.

Mindful Snacking: Keep healthy plant-based snacks on hand, like fresh fruit, veggie sticks, or air-popped popcorn.

Shop Seasonally: Purchase seasonal produce for better flavor and often lower prices.

Join a Community: Connect with local or online plant-based communities for recipe ideas and support.

4.2 Cooking Techniques and Substitutions

Plant-Based Proteins: Incorporate a variety of plant-based proteins such as legumes, tofu, tempeh, and seitan to ensure a well-balanced diet.

Grilling Vegetables: Enhance flavors by grilling vegetables like bell peppers, zucchini, and eggplant. It adds a smoky taste and retains nutrients.

Marinating Tofu: Marinate tofu in flavorful sauces or spices before cooking to infuse it with taste and improve its texture.

Crispy Roasting: Achieve a satisfying crunch by roasting vegetables at a high temperature. This method is great for Brussels sprouts, cauliflower, and sweet potatoes.

Substitute Dairy: Replace dairy in recipes with plant-based alternatives like almond milk, soy milk, or coconut milk for a creamy texture.
Flax or Chia Eggs: Use flax or chia seed gel as an egg substitute in baking. Mix 1 tablespoon of ground seeds with 3 tablespoons of water to replace one egg.

Nutritional Yeast: Add nutritional yeast to dishes for a cheesy flavor, providing a savory element to plant-based meals.

Homemade Vegetable Broth: Create a rich vegetable broth at home using vegetable scraps. It adds depth to soups, stews, and sauces.

Avocado in Baking: Swap butter with mashed avocado in baking for a healthier fat alternative that maintains moisture.

Lemon Zest: Use lemon zest to brighten up dishes. It adds a burst of flavor and acidity without extra calories.

Herb Infusions: Infuse oils or liquids with fresh herbs like rosemary, thyme, or basil to elevate the taste of your dishes.

Whole Grain Alternatives: Opt for whole grains like quinoa, brown rice, and barley instead of refined grains for added nutrients and fiber.

Vegetable Noodles: Replace traditional pasta with spiralized vegetables like zucchini or sweet potatoes for a low-carb alternative.

Cashew Cream: Make a creamy sauce using soaked and blended cashews for a dairy-free substitute in recipes like Alfredo or creamy soups.

Mindful Seasoning: Experiment with spices like cumin, paprika, turmeric, and nutritional yeast to enhance the flavors of your plant-based meals. Never forget that the greatest way to discover what suits your tastes is to try a variety of things.

CHAPTER FIVE

Maintaining a Plant-based Lifestyle Beyond 30 Days

Adopting a plant-based lifestyle goes beyond a 30-day challenge; it's a commitment to long-term health and environmental sustainability. In the initial month, individuals often experience physical and mental shifts as their bodies adapt to a plant-focused diet. However, the key to lasting success lies in incorporating variety, ensuring nutritional balance, and finding enjoyable plant-based recipes.

To maintain this lifestyle, education plays a pivotal role. Understanding the nutritional needs of a plant-based diet helps individuals make informed choices, ensuring they get essential nutrients like protein, iron, and B12. Planning meals ahead and exploring diverse plant-based sources, such as legumes, nuts, and seeds, contributes to a well-rounded diet.

Building a supportive community can be instrumental. Connecting with like-minded individuals provides a platform for sharing experiences, recipes, and tips. Additionally, staying informed about new plant-based products and cooking techniques keeps the lifestyle exciting and prevents monotony.

Flexibility is essential. Acknowledging that occasional deviations or adjustments may be necessary fosters a sustainable mindset. Whether for social reasons or personal preferences, allowing oneself flexibility prevents the diet from becoming a source of stress.

In essence, maintaining a plant-based lifestyle beyond 30 days involves continual learning, community support, and a flexible approach to ensure it becomes a lifelong, fulfilling choice.

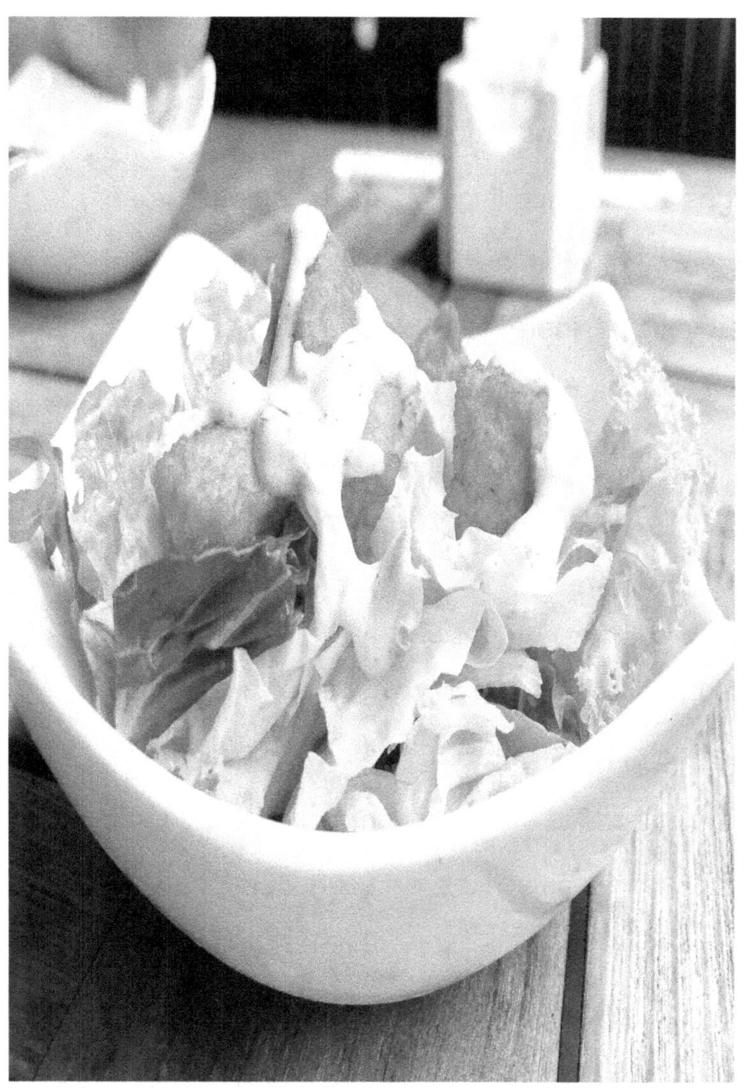

CHAPTER SIX

6 Conclusion

In conclusion, the adoption of a plant-based diet emerges as a compelling and sustainable approach to not only individual health but also environmental and ethical considerations. As we navigate the complexities of modern dietary choices, the shift towards plant-based eating stands out as a beacon of hope for a healthier, more environmentally conscious future.

Health benefits associated with a plant-based diet are manifold. Numerous studies have highlighted its potential to reduce the risk of chronic diseases such as heart disease, diabetes, and certain cancers. By embracing a diet rich in fruits, vegetables, whole grains, and legumes, individuals can harness the power of nature's nutrients to bolster their immune systems, maintain a healthy weight, and optimize overall well-being.

Moreover, the environmental implications of embracing plant-based eating cannot be overstated. The livestock industry is a major contributor to deforestation, water pollution, and greenhouse gas emissions. By choosing plant-based alternatives, individuals can actively participate in mitigating the environmental toll of animal agriculture. The conservation of natural resources and reduction of carbon footprints become tangible benefits of this dietary shift, contributing to the global effort to combat climate change.

Ethically, a plant-based diet aligns with the growing awareness of animal welfare issues. The industrialized methods of animal farming often involve cramped conditions, routine antibiotic use, and practices that raise ethical concerns. Opting for a plant-based lifestyle sends a powerful message in favor of compassion towards animals, promoting a more humane and sustainable approach to food production.

As we reflect on the advantages of a plant-based diet, it is crucial to acknowledge the importance of balance and informed choices. A well-planned plant-based diet can provide all essential nutrients, but attention to certain micronutrients, such as vitamin B12 and iron, is necessary. Consulting with healthcare professionals and nutrition experts can guide individuals in crafting a plant-based diet that meets their nutritional needs.

6.1 Reflections on the 30-day journey

Embarking on a 30-day plant-based diet journey has been transformative. Initially, I faced challenges adjusting to a new culinary landscape, but as days passed, I discovered a wealth of delicious and nutritious plant-based options. My energy levels surged, and I felt a sense of lightness in both body and conscience. The journey prompted me to explore diverse fruits, vegetables, and grains, expanding my palate and culinary skills.

Not only did I witness physical changes, like improved digestion and clearer skin, but there was a mental shift too. I became more mindful of my food choices and their impact on the environment. The ethical dimension of a plant-based lifestyle became increasingly apparent, aligning my diet with values of sustainability and compassion.

Navigating social situations posed occasional challenges, but the experience fostered resilience and creativity in finding plant-based alternatives. Connecting with a supportive community online provided valuable resources and encouragement.

As the 30 days concluded, I found myself contemplating a continued plant-based lifestyle. The journey not only reshaped my eating habits but also fostered a deeper connection to the broader ecosystem, promoting well-being and a harmonious coexistence with the planet.

6.2 Encouragement for a continued success

Embarking on a plant-based diet is a commendable journey towards a healthier, more sustainable lifestyle. As you embrace this path, remember that every small step contributes to your overall well-being and the well-being of the planet. The key to continued success lies in celebrating your achievements, no matter how modest they may seem.

Recognize the positive changes in your energy levels, mood, and perhaps even your physical appearance. Acknowledge the compassion you extend to animals and the positive impact on the environment by reducing your carbon footprint.

Embrace the learning process, experimenting with diverse plant-based foods to discover flavors and textures that delight your palate.

Surround yourself with a supportive community, whether it's friends, family, or online groups sharing similar journeys. Their encouragement and shared experiences can be invaluable in overcoming challenges and staying motivated. Additionally, stay informed about the nutritional aspects of a plant-based diet to ensure you meet your body's needs for essential nutrients.

Set realistic goals and milestones, celebrating each accomplishment along the way. Whether it's successfully incorporating more vegetables into your meals or finding a favorite plant-based recipe, these achievements propel you towards sustained success. Remember, it's not about perfection but progress.

53

Lastly, be kind to yourself. If you encounter setbacks, view them as opportunities to learn and adjust your approach. Cultivate a positive mindset, focusing on the joy and fulfillment that comes from nourishing your body with wholesome, plant-based foods. Your commitment to a plant-based lifestyle is a powerful investment in your health, the well-being of animals, and the sustainability of our planet. Keep thriving on this inspiring journey!

Daily meal repurposing

Day	Breakfast	Lunch	Dinner
Monday	Oatmeal	Chicken Salad	Spaghetti
Tuesday	Yogurt	Vegetabl	Grilled

55	Parfait	e Wrap	Salmon
Wednesday	Smoothie	Quinoa Bowl	Stir-Fry Vegetable
Thursday	Scrambled Eggs	Leftover Pizza	Chicken Stir-fry
Friday	Pancake	Tuna Salad	BBQ Chicken
Saturday	Avocado Toast	Turkey Sandwich	Pasta Primavera
Sunday	Fruit Salad	Rice and Beanseans	Grilled Vegetable